IN THIS MOMENT

The Art of Managing Stress Through Meditation

TERRY MALUK

CONTENTS

DEDICATION

To those who have always wanted to start meditating and didn't know how or weren't quite ready. May these words bring you motivation and confidence. Today's your day!

GIFT FROM TERRY

I understand how hard it can be to make time to be still or to try to be mindful while doing the many things in life. Now that you have your copy of *In This Moment*, you have what you need to create a calmer, more peaceful life through the simple practice of daily meditation. As you grow your practice, you'll begin to notice more ease and joy in your life.

As my gift to you, I've created an audio recording of a guided relaxation to accompany Chapter 1 as your first step to finding calm. In the **Notes** section near the back of this book you'll find a link where you can download your free copy.

Congratulations on taking this step. Enjoy the journey!

All the Best,

Terry

INTRODUCTION

She wondered aloud "Is this the day?"

And then she smiled,

knowing this was indeed the right moment to take the first step...

the first step, and the first smile, of many. – TM

Meditation has a profound impact on my life. It helps me go from scattered, stressed, and inefficient to more focused, calm, and peacefully productive. Since starting a regular meditation practice almost three decades ago, I am happier, more aware of what triggers stress and therefore less prone to react, and more mindful of everything that brings joy to my life.

I feel a genuine calm deep within. It takes something major to shake this core of peace, which is not to say I don't worry about this or that or get in a wad sometimes, because I do.

Instead of chaos and drama being a habitual way of life, I've learned to recognize when they arrive and to drop easily into my quiet and still center, at will, in a heartbeat, anytime.

As I witness myself successfully going within to regroup, I smile. I thank my meditation practice for giving me the ability to do this and so much more. My life is better because of meditation. It's that simple. I feel certain that my increased happiness contributes to a better quality of life for those around me as well. I want you to have this chance, too.

When you are able to become still and quiet your thinking mind each day, it will improve your life in so many ways... surprising ways you can't yet imagine.

A quick story... At the closing of my daily morning meditation, I silently ask what it is I need to know that day. Usually, a word comes to mind almost instantly, and most often the word is easy to understand based on what is going on in my life at the time. Words like "peace," "knowledge," "curiosity," "beauty" come to me. Easy, right? Some days I am given "patience," and I automatically wonder what will be coming that day. Usually, by the end of the evening, I smile as I recognize the significance of the word given to me that morning.

One day I was presented with a word for which I needed more clarification: "equanimity." I looked for a good definition, impressed that my subconscious, the Universe, my Higher Self, or whatever you may choose to call it, came up with something that wasn't totally clear. It helped me know it wasn't my thinking brain just making this stuff up each morning!

When I saw that equanimity meant remaining calm in difficult situations, I became a little concerned about what my day would offer. And by the end of that day I knew exactly why I was given that word. Between frequent breaks to be still, breathe, notice my feelings, or take a quick walk, I was able to maintain a sense of equanimity during a challenging day.

The ability to maintain a sense of calm and composure during one of life's rough spots is a treasure. Stress management tools, including meditation, can definitely help us come back to center, feel more grounded and level, better able to deal with the many opportunities that life offers.

I've been wanting to write a book on meditation for a long time, but when I started to do the research, I saw so many amazing books on meditation already available. Why would I want to add another one to the list? Why write about a topic that others have already offered in such beautiful ways?

These questions kept me stuck for a long time. Then I remembered I may have something different to offer that might reach even one person in exactly the way they need to hear it. Maybe I can offer a unique approach to this journey within. Perhaps I can do it in an easy and concise way that allows you to start from exactly where you are right now, *In This Moment*.

This book is for those who are new to meditation, curious, and may be ready to give it a try. It is also for those familiar with some form of meditation practice who are perhaps seeking a new beginning. It is for anyone who brings the wonderful gift of an open, receptive mind to this journey.

In this book, you'll start right away with a guided relaxation meditation so you can easily experience the benefits of a meditation practice. From there, you'll read about some of the definitions of meditation, what it is and what it is not, and learn about many of the reasons to develop a regular practice. Then you'll get to learn and experience a variety of meditation practices, including meditating on the breath, meditating with kindness, practicing meditation while in nature and while walking, gratitude meditation, and guided yoga nidra meditation. Finally, you'll read some suggestions on how to make meditation a habit for good. Spoiler alert... practice, practice, practice!

Several references from the very large body of research on using meditation to reduce stress, bring calm, control anger, lower blood pressure, ease pain, increase happiness, ease depression and more, are included in the Notes section. Some of the words in this book are adapted from portions of my other books: *Rx for RNs: A Step-by-Step Guide to Manage Stress, Reduce Overwhelm, and Conquer Burnout*, which includes other stress management techniques in addition to meditation, and *Take One Breath: The Art of Managing Stress Through Mindful Breathing*.

For the first time, I'm sharing some of my original poetry with you at the start of each chapter. I hope you like them! There is also one poem at the beginning of Chapter 2, too perfect to not include, from an unknown author.

Ready to start? Take a slow, comforting breath, and know you are exactly where you need to be.

Please remember: It's important to contact a professional if things feel too big for you. Never discontinue current medications without first consulting your doctor.

GUIDED RELAXATION
MEDITATION

Lost in thought,

not here in this moment,

instead elsewhere,

wandering in the familiar past or possible futures,

missing the precious present

and its beauty.

Look up.

You are here. – TM

Many people mention that they want to start a meditation practice but haven't gotten around to it or didn't know how to begin. Perhaps you are reading this now because starting a meditation practice is on your list of intentions and goals to improve your life.

Congratulations on taking this step! Meditation is easy to practice, costs little to nothing, and is straightforward to learn.

QUICKSTART TO MEDITATION: GUIDED RELAXATION

One of the easiest ways to get started is to listen to a short, guided relaxation audio that will leave you feeling more calm and peaceful. This can be the perfect introduction to meditation because your only tasks are to get comfortable, listen, and allow the magic of relaxation to happen. Once you experience how even a short practice like this can help you feel better quickly, you'll be ready to make meditation a habit for good.

Begin by downloading your free seven-minute guided relaxation audio that accompanies this chapter. You'll find the link in the Notes section near the back of this book.[1]

Becoming still and listening to a guided relaxation is a great way to begin your day and an easy way to unwind and release stress at the end of the day so you can fall asleep more easily. If time allows, try practicing both in the morning and in the evening.

By treating yourself to guided relaxation recordings, you begin to increase your awareness of yourself, your environment, and your feelings. You'll experience the sense of peace that comes with releasing the stress of daily life. With regular practice, you'll learn to more easily recognize your reactions to stress so you can better control them in the moment and gain confidence in your ability to manage stress at any time.

Once you've experienced this relaxing start to your journey, it's time to learn more about meditation, starting with what meditation is, what it is not, and some of the many benefits you'll receive from a regular practice.

ENHANCE YOUR PRACTICE

You can make meditation a special gift to yourself by scheduling an appointment on your calendar. I highly recommend that you set aside this time so you won't be disturbed, when there's nothing else you need to be doing and nowhere else you need to be. In this way, you'll fully experience the benefits of a guided relaxation meditation.

Knowing that your schedule is probably over-booked, I promise that setting these seven minutes aside for self-care will reward your effort. Set your wake-up alarm for ten minutes early or find ten minutes before falling asleep to listen. Enjoy!

❧ 2 ❧
WHY MEDITATE?

"It's impossible," said pride.

"It's risky," said experience.

"It's pointless," said reason.

"Give it a try," whispered the heart. – Author Unknown

My first answer to the question "Why meditate?" is another question: "Why NOT meditate?"

Addressing the points in the above quote, a meditation practice is definitely possible and can even be easy. Risky? The only risk is becoming aware of and learning to appreciate yourself and the world around you. Meditation is far from pointless, as you experienced in Chapter 1. So why not give it a try? The heart offers excellent advice.

In this chapter, I'll cover a few of the most frequently asked questions about what meditation is, briefly address what meditation is not, and then list some of the many benefits of meditation along with references to resources containing further information.

WHAT MEDITATION IS

Merriam-Webster suggests that meditation is a noun. It's defined as "The act or process of spending time in quiet thought: the act or process of meditating."[1]

According to Yogapedia, "Meditation is the process of quieting the mind in order to spend time in thought for relaxation or religious/spiritual purposes. The goal is to attain an inner state of awareness and intensify personal and spiritual growth."[2]

The Cambridge Dictionary says meditation is "The act of giving your attention to only one thing, either as a religious activity or as a way of becoming calm and relaxed."[3]

Meditation is easy to practice. It's free, and there are very few rules, if any, about how to practice. You can try it almost anywhere without special props, postures, clothes, music, chanting, incense, or any of the other things people often associate with meditation.

Meditation has been practiced in parts of the world for thousands of years. While archeologists and scholars agree that it has been practiced for about five thousand years, written records about meditation were discovered around 1500 BCE. It wasn't until the 18th century that translations began to make their way to Western scholars.

Many books have been written about various forms of meditation and how the practice has evolved over time. However, until recently, it was considered too "out there" in many people's minds to be seriously considered. Enter well-known authors such as Wayne Dyer, Deepak Chopra, Eckhart Tolle, Jon Kabat-Zinn, Sharon Salzberg, and many others, to help Western minds better understand the idea that a meditation practice can greatly improve the quality of life.

Meditation has become a mainstream topic as more and more people take the opportunity to learn about meditation and its benefits. Many research articles, blog posts, podcasts, and books describe what meditation is and offer definitions of the word. These definitions vary widely by source, some even contradicting one another, but one common theme is that meditation is the act of quieting our thoughts so that awareness of the present moment can be experienced and expanded.

There are likely as many types of meditation practices as there are practitioners, each of us customizing variations on a theme to find what works best for us in each moment. My hope is that by directly experiencing the range of practices presented in this book, you'll have a better idea of what meditation is and how you can best fit a regular practice into your life.

What is meditation for me? My daily practice has made a huge difference in my life since I started all those year ago. For me, meditation brings me joy and allows me to remain calmer and more centered than I would be without it.

My current personal practice begins with a seated morning meditation of differing lengths spent in silence or listening to a guided audio. I focus on enjoying the day with an open awareness of *what is* from moment to moment as best I can, including my feelings, emotions, and my surroundings. I close my day with evening meditation in the form of quiet contemplation and a written gratitude practice.

This is definitely not *the* way to meditate for anyone else. It is *one* way that works for me right now and it may change tomorrow. Meditation is different for everyone, which makes perfect sense since we are all beautifully unique individuals.

WHAT MEDITATION IS NOT

Some sources suggest meditation is something to be afraid of for various reasons. Many let this fear mentality keep them from learning about and trying meditation. Here are just a few of the things that meditation is often claimed to be but in reality, is not.

Meditation is not a religion, nor does meditation replace religion. While many religions include meditation as part of their traditions, meditation itself is *not* a religion. Nor does one need to practice any particular religion or be a "religious" person to practice meditation.

Meditation is not a ritual associated with any single culture or group.

Meditation is not meant only for those seeking a more spiritual life. It is for everyone.

Meditation is not a form of mind control. Rather than trying to control, meditation is more about relaxing, observing, and letting go of thoughts, allowing the mind to become comfortable with being still and quiet.

Meditation is not a form of self-hypnosis.

Meditation is not difficult to practice.

Meditation is not unattainable. Many people experience a sort of peaceful calm at some point in their lives without even trying, often in a quiet natural setting. This is similar to states achieved during meditation. If you tried the guided audio in Chapter 1, you already know meditation is attainable.

THE BENEFITS OF MEDITATION

There are many benefits of having a meditation practice. It is a well-accepted method to manage stress, and that's what this book is all about. Scientific studies show that with regular practice, meditation reduces stress in the short term and provides a long-term stress buffer effect. This means that, faced with your most common daily stressors, you won't react as quickly or strongly. You're better able to choose and direct your response.

With reduced stress, you also neutralize feelings such as worry, fear, anxiety, tension, and even blood pressure issues. As you create a daily meditation practice, you invite and allow feelings of calm, joy, and peace to fill your life. And you can experience this benefit quickly and easily. All you need to do is be still and take a few breaths with awareness.

Many studies show, not surprisingly, that meditation can also reduce the many effects of chronic stress on the body. Research shows that immune and endocrine measures of inflammation and stress are significantly lower in those who practice mindfulness-based stress reduction (MBSR),[4] where mindfulness is the state of being aware of what is happening in the present moment.

A 2014 meta-analysis of over six hundred research papers found that meditation is more effective than most alternative treatments for anxiety, and that results were positively correlated with the level of stress and anxiety.[5] This means that the more stressed or anxious you are, the better meditation works to provide relief.

One randomized control study looked at the effect of using MBSR on health care professionals. The results showed reduced stress and an increase in quality of life and self-compassion among the study participants.[6] In other words, work-related stress can be relieved through meditation.

Another benefit of mindfulness meditation is how it helps you become aware of how you feel, your surroundings, and the choices you have. A 2012 study shows the practice of mindfulness meditation allows the brain to more creatively process. "The authors conclude that mindfulness meditation reduces cognitive rigidity via the tendency to be 'blinded' by experience. Results are discussed in light of the benefits of mindfulness practice regarding a reduced tendency to over-look novel and adaptive ways of responding due to past experience, both in and out of the clinical setting."[7] This means you can stop reacting mindlessly to a familiar situation based on past behaviors and use your creative brain to find a better response.

By practicing meditation regularly, you train your brain to maintain focus, thus lengthening your attention span. A longer attention span means you can stay on task longer and, with practice, more easily notice when you're not on task. Further, you develop a greater ability to reorient back to the task if you've wandered off course. This is a significant benefit in the age of attention deficit.[8]

A study of human resource workers showed that "the meditation group reported lower levels of stress and showed better memory for the tasks they had performed; they also switched tasks less often and remained focused on tasks longer."[9] Other studies have shown meditation helps to reduce age-related memory loss, increase positive feelings and actions toward the self and others, may help fight addictions by increasing self-control and self-awareness of triggers for addictive behaviors, and decrease blood pressure.

Another huge benefit of meditation is improved sleep. Many of the people with whom I work initially complain of some type of sleep disorder. Statistics show that almost half of the population suffer from lack of sleep. Meditation reduces stress, which reduces insomnia. In a study of the effect of meditation on sleep, participants who meditated fell asleep sooner and stayed asleep longer, compared to those who didn't meditate.[10] When you sleep better, life is better for you and everyone around you.

Meditation can help reduce and relieve pain. A few minutes spent calming the mind helps the muscles in the body to relax thereby reducing physical and mental tension. When you can relax, pain will usually decrease and may even disappear completely. It's all connected. Research shows that meditators reported less sensitivity to pain and showed increased activity in the brain centers known to control pain.[11]

Meditation increases awareness, not just self-awareness, but also of your surroundings. Awareness brings new skills to the table. Once you begin to recognize the triggers and first signs of stress and anxiety, you can take pre-emptive steps to avoid the downward spiral of stress-induced behaviors.

Meditation allows clarity. As you become still and focus on nothing at all, or perhaps watch your breathing, the mind chatter quiets. Okay, maybe not in the first minute... but once you settle into your practice, all the chaos that normally fills your mind begins to settle, like particles settle in a lake after the rain stops. You are able to see a little deeper, and deeper yet, to the still point beneath the surface. Sitting with that quiet, still point, the answers to questions you've been mulling over or solutions to problems you've been facing will appear without even trying.

Meditation helps you smile. Sometimes during my morning meditation, as I quiet my thoughts and sit in silence, ideas will come, or I'll realize something that should have been obvious, but I wasn't seeing it until that moment. And I smile, because it had been there the whole time. I was simply too distracted to see it. As clarity comes with stillness, that in itself brings happiness.

This list is just a sample of the many benefits of a meditation practice. Many more research findings are being published almost daily proving the benefits of meditation.[12] Since you now know how helpful it can be for so many things, this is a great time to commit to developing a daily practice.

There is so much more about meditation to learn and experience. This list is enough to help you get started. I've spent decades practicing, learning, and benefiting from meditation and, with my whole heart, I recommend you give it a try.

ENHANCE YOUR PRACTICE

When you're ready to take your solo meditation practice further, there are several good, free meditation apps for Android and iPhone such as Insight Timer, Headspace, and Stop, Breathe & Think. If you still consider yourself a meditation doubter, check out the 10% Happier app created specifically for the skeptic. You can also find other apps that require a fee to access. For group practice, check with local yoga studios or Meetup groups in your area.

ॐ 3 ॐ

MEDITATE ON THE BREATH

Breathing in, my body senses the silent change

as the last soft, warm air of afternoon

surrenders to the first cool, crisp air of evening. – TM

Being led through a guided relaxation, such as you experienced in Chapter 1, is one of the easiest ways to meditate. Guided relaxation introduces you to the concept of becoming still, paying attention, and becoming mindful through guided focus on one thing at a time.

Focusing solely on the breath is probably the next easiest way to meditate, as this provides awareness of the natural connection between mind and body. Many breathing meditations are based on the ancient yogic technique of *pranayama*, a Sanskrit term roughly translated to mean control of the breath.

According to the *Yoga Sutras* of Patanjali[1], *pranayama* is the fourth of the eight limbs of yoga that, when practiced regularly, can help us become more aware of how we feel and help us relax and release negative feelings.

Meditative breathing, says meditation master Thich Nhat Hanh, is a tool to calm the mind so it can see into itself and gain insight that can lead to a state of enlightenment. Using the breath as a focal point not only strengthens the ability of the mind to concentrate, it also stimulates compassion, awakening our true nature.[2]

There are dozens of breathing techniques that are useful for a meditation practice. Five of them are covered in the first book in this series called *Take One Breath: The Art of Managing Stress Through Mindful Breathing*, including heart breathing, abdominal breathing, and ocean breathing.

In this chapter, you'll experience a simple method of breathing with awareness by counting while you breathe, thereby giving the mind something on which to concentrate to help calm racing thoughts. Next, moving on to a deeper state of noticing the subtle aspects of breathing, you'll become familiar with how it feels to free yourself from what is often called the monkey mind.

Keep in mind that the right breathing meditation is the one that works for you. As you try each one in this chapter and find yourself returning to one in particular, that's your practice, at least in this moment. As life happens, you may find a different practice better suits your needs. Trust your heart and your breath to know what's right for you.

As the Exploration of Consciousness (EOC) Research Institute shares, "In his classic guide to meditation practice, *Wherever You Go, There You Are*, Jon Kabat-Zinn writes this about breathing: 'It helps to have a focus for your attention, an anchor line to tether you to the present moment and to guide you back when the mind wanders. The breath serves this purpose... Bringing awareness to our breathing we remind ourselves that we are here now.'"[3] Mindful breathing can be a quick and powerful way to bring us back to center.

Breathing meditations can be practiced in almost any posture. If you have time and the setting allows, practice while sitting or reclining comfortably. A bedtime breathing meditation practice can help ease you into sleep. You can practice a short breathing meditation if you wake up in the middle of the night to help you get back to sleep, and a one-minute breathing practice first thing as you awaken can keep your mind from taking off in a million directions before you've even hit the ground. You can also practice while walking or standing. For example, while on your way to a stressful task or meeting, taking a few slow, calming breaths on the way can help you arrive with more focus and clarity.

4-7-8 BREATHING

Dr. Andrew Weil has made popular the 4-7-8 Breath, also known as the Relaxing Breath, as an easy way to manage stress and help you find relaxation almost immediately.[4] This technique becomes a calming meditation once you become familiar and comfortable with the counting pattern. The pattern might, at first, seem complex and uncomfortable, but with only a little practice the breathing pattern quickly becomes more natural and soothing. Soon you will no longer need to concentrate on the counting and a meditative relaxation happens.

The practice of 4-7-8 breathing can take place anywhere and anytime, making it super easy to use exactly when you need it. Initially, you may wish to set aside a little time to become familiar with the counting pattern and how it feels in your body.

Dr. Weil suggests keeping the tip of your tongue just behind your upper teeth while practicing the 4-7-8 Breath, and there are others who practice 4-7-8 breathing with a relaxed tongue. You can try it both ways and notice which method relaxes you more.

The 4-7-8 Breath starts after an exhalation, with empty lungs:

- Inhale through your nose to a count of **four**.
- Next hold your full breath for a count of **seven**.
- Then purse your lips and exhale forcefully through the mouth to a count of **eight**, making a whooshing sound as you empty the lungs.

That's one breath. You're now back to the beginning with empty lungs and ready to start the next breath by inhaling through your nose to a count of four. By exhaling for twice as long as you inhale, you initiate the relaxation response in the body.

Take four breaths like this so that you begin to feel at ease with the counting and breathing rhythm. Practice using the 4-7-8 pattern for four breaths twice each day for four to six weeks and notice how much easier it becomes. Seriously, put it on your schedule twice a day at a convenient time for you. It only takes one minute of your time twice a day. Is it worth two minutes of your day to feel more relaxed all the time?

Once you are comfortable with the technique, you may begin noticing times during your day where you start the 4-7-8 Breath automatically to help you find calm during a stressful moment. It is recommended that you do no more than eight breath cycles at a time.

Easy, right? Inhale through your nose to four, hold for seven, exhale through your mouth to eight. Adjust the pace of your breathing and counting until you are comfortable holding your full breath for a count of seven. Some benefits of the 4-7-8 Breath include reduced stress and anxiety, improved digestion, lower blood pressure, and better control of cravings.

COUNTING EACH BREATH

Another way of counting while breathing as a form of meditation involves counting each inhalation and exhalation, starting at one and progressing to ten. Stop when you notice the mind has wandered and start again at one. This practice is all about noticing how the mind can easily jump from where you are and what you are doing to the other things going on in your life.

Start by finding a comfortable position, either sitting or reclining. Allow yourself to settle in so you have no distractions. If you'd like to set a timer for five or ten minutes so you don't need to worry about the time, do that first. Allow your eyes to close if that's comfortable or focus on a chosen object such as a flower or picture or candle.

Breathing normally, begin counting your breaths to yourself. On an inhalation, say to yourself "Inhaling. One." And on the exhalation say to yourself "Exhaling. One." Then "Inhaling. Two. Exhaling. Two." Continue counting while you inhale and exhale until you reach ten. If you like, you can begin again. Or if your mind has wandered, and it will, start over at one on your next inhalation.

When you notice the mind has wandered, rather than judging yourself and your monkey mind, celebrate the noticing because this is a huge step. So often the mind races invisibly in the background, keeping you from being fully present. By learning to notice this tendency, you can smile and practice returning your focus to patiently counting each breath.

Once you are comfortable counting each part of the breath, you can simplify this type of meditation by saying to yourself, slowly, "Inhaling... and exhaling... one." Continue counting this way until you reach ten, starting over when the mind has wandered. You'll notice that the more you practice, the less frequently the mind will wander. As you settle, so will the mind.

INHALING WHAT YOU DESIRE

As a different focus, you can use the steady rhythm of your inhale as a meditation to invite and allow more of what you desire into your life, and then exhale what you're ready to release. This is a surprisingly powerful and fun variation. In addition to the relaxation response from a regular breathing meditation practice, this "in with the good and out with the bad" focus is uplifting and freeing, bringing hope, joy, and a more positive outlook.

It's very simple to inhale what you desire. Find a comfortable position and settle in if you prefer a quiet, distraction-free practice, or use this technique anytime you want to feel better, such as driving down the road or waiting in a line.

Decide on something you'd like to invite into your life. Examples might be peace, joy, happiness, clarity, patience, health, or some other positive feeling or thing. Then decide what negative aspect you are ready to release. Examples might be fear, anger, frustration, shame, worry, or stress. Choose several if they come to mind.

Once you've identified your words, slowly begin to deepen and lengthen each inhalation and release the breath slowly. Let yourself find a comfortably deep breathing rhythm. Then, on an inhale, say to yourself, "Inhaling peace." On your exhale, say to yourself, "Exhaling stress." Substitute these sample words with what is right for you each time you practice. Either set a timer for five or ten minutes or allow yourself to breathe until you feel you've invited and released enough.

As with all practices, notice how you feel after inhaling what you desire and exhaling what you don't. Adjust your words as more ideas arise and you become more comfortable with the practice.

THE NEXT STAGES OF A BREATHING MEDITATION

After practicing for a week or two while counting the breath, and when it feels right for you, let the counting fall away completely so that you are only observing the breath. This takes a little more dedication because, without the helpful focal point of counting, the mind may feel free to slip away, and it will. Gently bring it back to noticing each inhalation and exhalation, each breath as it comes and goes.

You might wonder what there is to notice about breathing. Here are just a few things to pay attention to:

- Become aware of the temperature of the air being inhaled. Is the air cool in your nostrils?
- As you exhale, is the air leaving your body a little warmer?
- How far do you feel the air move into your body?

Where do you feel it? In the back of your throat or down into your chest?

- Notice if the chest or belly rise as you inhale and how everything releases back down as you exhale.
- Maybe there's a little space of time between the inhale and exhale that you can observe and explore.
- On your next exhalation, can you empty every bit of air out?
- At the end of your exhalations, are you still for a nanosecond before the next inhalation? Does your mind and body become completely still in that moment?
- Consider how it feels to lengthen and deepen each breath.
- Notice how it feels to bring your breathing back to normal.
- Appreciate how you feel after breathing with so much awareness.

Taking your breathing meditation one step further, let go of noticing the process of breathing. Let yourself relax. While breathing normally, see if you can focus on the subtle sensations at the tip of your nose. Notice how the breath feels coming in and going out of the tip of your nose. Take five very slow, comfortably deep breaths while maintaining this narrower focus. Notice if your mind wanders more or less using this focus. Either way, congratulate yourself on your efforts.

ENHANCE YOUR PRACTICE

During any meditation practice, things happen. Dogs bark, phones ring, environments change, monkey mind comes back... don't give up! This is an excellent way to train yourself to handle interruptions both during meditation and in the rest of your day.

If your meditation becomes distracted by random thoughts, acknowledge them and simply say to yourself, "Thinking," and come back to your focus. If you begin to feel hot, cold, or some other sensation, acknowledge it and say to yourself, "Sensation," and come back to your focus. If your meditation is interrupted by noises, acknowledge them and say to yourself, "Hearing," and come back to your focus.

Use a one-word neutral description of whatever is going on that causes you to lose your focus and then come right back to your focus. These distractions are normal and natural, and coming back to focus gets much easier with practice.

In all these variations of meditating on the breath, please remember to breathe slowly enough so you don't feel light-headed. And after each practice, when you return to your normal breathing, notice how you feel. People often report feeling lighter, calmer, more relaxed yet energized, and more joyful.

Use these quick and easy meditations to release, relieve, and reduce stress while increasing mindfulness and awareness. See which ones work best for you and allow yourself to develop a daily practice. You'll be glad you did.

彩 4 彩

MEDITATE WITH KINDNESS

With an open heart,

receiving and sending,

love, kindness, and compassion.

I savor the gift and the giving. – TM

According to expert Sharon Salzberg[1], co-founder of the Insight Meditation Society, offering feelings of goodwill, kindness, and warmth toward ourselves and others as a meditation practice is called *metta* meditation, or loving-kindness meditation. This type of meditation can be an easy practice for some and a more challenging practice for others. Sending out good vibes to ourselves is one thing. Sending those same good thoughts out to people towards whom we have negative feelings can be difficult at first.

Wishes can be general such as offering love, peace, kindness, health, or compassion, or they can be unique to each intended recipient. The wishes may also be specific, such as for relief from physical pain or freedom from negative situations like danger or hunger.

Over time, a loving-kindness meditation practice is very relaxing and rewarding. If it's not your favorite meditation style when you first try it, give it two weeks and see how you feel. There are many other meditation styles if it turns out this one just doesn't feel good to you.

BENEFITS OF PRACTICING LOVING-KINDNESS

Research has shown that practicing loving-kindness meditation has a wide range of benefits. In addition to helping us feel good during the practices themselves, our overall sense of well-being is enhanced, helping us to become more positive and satisfied with life. We feel connected to the world by sending out those good wishes, which can lead to an increased sense of purpose.[2]

There are many studies reporting on the benefits of loving-kindness meditation, as seen in a summary article from *Psychology Today*,[3] from increases in positive emotions and decreases in negative emotions, to decreased migraines, chronic pain[4], PTSD symptoms and negative bias towards others, to increased empathy and social connections.

Used in the classroom as part of mindfulness training, a regular loving-kindness meditation practice for seven minutes each day was shown to reduce implicit racial bias.[5] It helps both students and teachers replace their automatic, unconscious thoughts about others with mindfully chosen new ways of acting and reacting.

PUTTING LOVING-KINDNESS INTO PRACTICE

When first starting your loving-kindness meditation practice, I recommend listening to a guided audio so that you get comfortable with the process. The guided audios come in a variety of lengths to choose from so you can match the time you have available. There are a few recommendations near the end of this chapter.

As you listen to more of them, you may have a favorite voice you enjoy. You may enjoy using guided loving-kindness meditations exclusively so that you don't have to think about how to do it or what to say next and you can be more fully in touch with the kindness you are offering.

The practice starts with offering yourself well-wishes before expanding your focus outward to a person for whom you have kind feelings or who has been kind to you. Next, the focus is on one person or more with whom you have a neutral experience... neither good nor bad. From there, the focus is on someone with whom you have had a bad experience and finally, opening up the offer of loving-kindness to all beings.

If you are practicing on your own, the words can be generic or they can be specific to the person or group receiving your intention of loving-kindness. Below is an example of a loving-kindness meditation, so that you know what to expect when listening to a guided audio.

Find a comfortable seated or reclined position in a place where you won't be disturbed. Use soothing background music if you like. Take a few slow, comfortably deep breaths to settle in and begin to quiet the mind and body. Bring your focus to your heart. Imagine being able to inhale abundant love into your heart and able to exhale love and kindness, compassion, and caring.

Start with directing the loving-kindness wishes toward yourself. This may feel awkward at first, but keep trying, using words such as:

May I be happy, safe, and calm.
May I be free from suffering.
May my heart be open and loving.
May I find peace and joy each day.

And, of course, if you have specific words of intention for yourself, include them.

Next, while thinking of someone special to you or someone for whom you have positive feelings, repeat the same words or use words that apply to that person. This part of the meditation may be the easiest for you:

May you be happy, safe, and calm.
May you be free from suffering.
May your heart be open and loving.
May you find peace and joy each day.

Moving on to a neutral person towards whom you have neither positive nor negative feelings, repeat using similar words or use words more specific to them:

May you be happy, safe, and calm.
May you be free from suffering.
May your heart be open and loving.
May you find peace and joy each day.

Now stretching yourself a bit, offer words of loving-kindness to someone towards whom you have negative feelings. This could be someone with whom you've had an argument or even someone in the news you don't care for. Use the same words above or choose words specifically for this person, remembering to keep the intention of loving-kindness and not let any negative feelings creep into your words:

May you be happy, safe, and calm.
May you be free from suffering.
May your heart be open and loving.
May you find peace and joy each day.

Think about this for a moment. How much better would everyone involved feel if this person really was feeling happy, safe, and calm? What if they had no suffering? What if their hearts were open and joyful and they felt surrounded by loving-kindness? Perhaps then they wouldn't be causing others to have negative feelings toward them. This thought can make it easier during this portion of the practice.

And finally, move your attention to include all beings, everyone on the planet, all living things, plants and animals, including yourself:

May we each be happy, safe, and calm.
May we each be free from suffering.
May our hearts be open and loving.
May we each find peace and joy each day.

After these rounds of loving-kindness, take three slow, comfortably deep breaths to finish your practice. Notice how you feel. There is no right or wrong feeling here. You will likely feel a little different after each practice; take the time to notice that. Sometimes the practice is totally fulfilling, and you'll want to take an extra minute or so to savor that feeling.

Other times it seems more mechanical, like you are simply going through the motions. But it's all good.

Here are a few free guided audios to help you get started. Or use your favorite search engine to find your own.

- Guided Loving-Kindness Meditation from Sharon Salzberg (46 minutes): https://www.mindful.org/loving-kindness-takes-time-sharon-salzberg/
- Loving-Kindness Meditation from Tara Brach (22 minutes): https://www.tarabrach.com/guided-meditation-loving-kindness/
- Loving-Kindness Meditation from Greater Good in Action at Berkeley University (14 minutes): https://ggia.berkeley.edu/practice/loving_kindness_meditation

∿

ENHANCE YOUR PRACTICE

Show yourself a little love and self-care by taking five minutes each day to practice offering yourself loving kindness. This can be such an uplifting practice that you'll look forward to it each day. Put one or both hands over your heart, or just imagine yourself with your hands over your heart. Take a slow, comfortably deep breath in as you imagine inhaling a sparkling white light representing love and well wishes to yourself. As you exhale, imagine the white light filling every cell in your whole body.

Take at least five breaths in this manner as you feel yourself beginning to glow. You can offer yourself forgiveness, courage, strength, gratitude, and anything else you need that day. Carry this light with you throughout your day.

MEDITATE IN NATURE

July's whisper-soft pink blossoms

blanket the Blue Ridge trails.

The rhododendron hover protectively over the warm orange lilies

as they shyly peek out to share their beauty.

Pockets of bright red celebrations of bee balm demand my gaze

as I wander,

beckoning me to slow my pace.

I breathe in this gift of nature's color and grace. – TM

---

editating in nature is an easy way to reconnect with all the senses in the body while allowing the mind to settle into stillness. There's a reason people are drawn to the park benches under a tree or near the water. It's a natural tendency to want to be surrounded by what the great outdoors offers, be it the sights, sounds, smells, or enjoying the feel of the air on your skin.

Most people have access to some piece of nature. It may be a small patch of green in the town square, a view of the sky from a window, or a large expanse of forest, desert, or ocean to wander through or alongside. Giving in to the call to linger in an outdoor setting is good for the soul and can help you find awareness and a unique type of meditation practice.

BENEFITS OF MEDITATING IN NATURE

I remember once, when I was quite young, hiking on a new trail in the lush forest of North Carolina. I took a break to sit on a boulder. It was the first time I ever sat still in nature. Soon the silence and stillness surrounded me, like a soft, protective hug.

I lost myself in the sights and sounds and smells of this place. I found connection with something much greater than myself. I experienced a profound sense of peace and well-being that I had never known before. I sat for longer than I intended, soaking up the feeling. This was my introduction to meditation, and it has been a love affair ever since.

Many retreats and workshops of all kinds are held in natural settings. Most monasteries are located in forests, surrounded by lush beauty and silence from man's constant commotion. These centers know the benefits of being in nature.

Meditating in open air can help you find relief from your day-to-day stress more quickly than your practice space at home. There's something about being surrounded by nature that allows us to more quickly feel calm.

Nature provides the perfect background sounds for practicing awareness. You can make the music of nature your focus, listening to the constant background harmonies, then noticing the intermittent tones of the wind in the trees, birdsong, or rustling of leaves. This moving target of focus allows the mind freedom to bounce around a bit, while maintaining attention exactly where you are in this moment.

According to psychotherapist, author, and meditation teacher Mark Coleman, meditating outside helped him feel "more wakeful and alert and, at the same time, open, relaxed, and spacious."[1,2]

Outdoor meditation improves mental health, reduces stress and anxiety, and thereby provides a variety of health benefits.[3] As stress is reduced, blood pressure decreases. It's all connected! In addition to outdoor meditation, exercising outdoors can also yield meditative benefits. Activities such as yoga, tai chi, or chi gong, when practiced outside, are especially rewarding and beneficial.

If possible, allow yourself to enjoy the direct contact of your bare feet on the ground. According to Mindworks, a mindfulness meditation app, when we are directly touching the ground, "our body's rhythm synchronizes with the earth's natural vibrations. This harmony greatly enhances the experience of meditation."[4]

There is a practice that began in Japan called "forest bathing,"[5] which is the practice of walking slowly through a forest while enjoying all the sensory input. Researcher and physician Quin Li reports that more and more people are suffering from "nature deficit disorder" due to spending an increasing amount of time indoors.

Dr. Li's book, *Forest Bathing: How Trees Can Help You Find*

Health and Happiness,[6] points out many of the benefits of being outdoors. After years of study, he reports the benefits of spending time in a forest include decreased stress, anxiety, depression, and anger. A slow walking meditation through a forest also strengthens the immune system and improves sleep, cardiovascular, and metabolic health.

PRACTICING MEDITATION IN NATURE

To practice forest bathing, all you need to do is find a patch of green. Hopefully there is at least a small park that is convenient. Some people are lucky enough to have large, wooded yards.

Dr. Li says walking under evergreen trees is especially beneficial, but you don't need to go miles into a forest to have a good practice. Once you are there, take a slow, comfortably deep breath and release it just as slowly. As you walk, take your time and let all your senses awaken to what's happening around you. Let your awareness sharpen to even the most subtle sensory input.

If you have extra time, sit, be still, and breathe. Soak in the silence or the unique forest sounds. You could even bring lunch to enjoy while in the forest. If you're a writer, this might be a perfect place for creative inspiration; channel your inner Emerson or Thoreau! If you like to take pictures, play with lighting and composition and enjoy all the colors of green the forest offers. You may feel drawn to touch the bark of a particular tree. Notice the texture and how it feels to place your palm on it. However you choose to experience this patch of nature, allow yourself to be fully absorbed in it.

Another common place to meditate in nature is the beach. While some beaches may be a bit crowded, I prefer finding a quieter section where I can both walk and sit. A slow walk along the shoreline can be a meditation itself, or finding a place to sit, listening to the waves, enjoying the smell of salt air, and allowing the gaze to soften as you watch the horizon. Try to tune out any man-made noise and bring your focus to the sounds and sight of the waves. Breathe.

Staying with the water theme, creeks, rivers, and waterfalls also provide great environments for outdoor meditation. You can become hypnotized by the random movements of the water, soften your gaze to a wider focus, or close your eyes and let yourself be surrounded by the changing sounds. Let your awareness tune in to your focal point and feel your stress melt away.

While meditating indoors can provide more of an internal centering, meditating outdoors can actually be easier as you allow your awareness to expand beyond your body or the breath. Once you choose an external focus for your meditation, which could be sights, sounds, or textures, try not to get caught up in *thinking* about it. That's the tricky part. Be aware of the sensory input without judgment. Release any stories about it that your mind wants to create. Notice the mind is thinking and then come back to your focus. Celebrate that you noticed!

WALKING MEDITATION

Another option for your meditation practice in nature is walking. This practice takes a little more practice when you first start because there is so much going on with your body in motion as well as continually changing sensory input from the environment. The benefit of this challenge is that you learn to adapt your still, quiet, seated practice to the world you inhabit each day. This is a huge accomplishment. When you can learn to be centered, calm, and focused during your day-to-day activities, your life becomes richer, easier, and more joyful.

You can start a walking meditation practice simply, finding a short path on which to learn the process. At first, your concentration can be on each small part of the physical mechanics of walking, noticing the feelings as you lift one foot slowly, bring it forward, then noticing as each different part of the foot makes contact with the ground, as the back foot begins to lift up, as your weight shifts forward, as the back foot leaves the ground, as the back leg moves toward the mid-line and then forward, then as each part of that foot touches the ground, and so on.[7]

There is also the upper body activity to notice. Your arms may swing a bit, your torso may move forward, backward or side-to-side to maintain balance as you progress. Your head may bow forward as your eyes scan the ground for objects to avoid on your next step, then back up again as you look forward. Your hearing is heightened as you listen for others on foot or bicycles.

Learning to notice the many subtleties of walking outside takes practice and gives you a new appreciation for this amazing set of coordinated, almost automatic movements. Adding awareness of the breath as you walk, perhaps finding a pattern of inhalations and exhalations to match your steps, helps you maintain focus.

Once you've practiced noticing what happens when you walk, you'll be able to increase your speed a little while still noticing. This allows you to take your practice further along your path, both literally and figuratively, as you grow your meditation practice out into the world.

A classic resource for learning about walking meditation is author Thich Nhat Hanh. He reminds us to take each step with reverence, no matter where we are walking. When we walk with mindfulness, it helps us be present in this moment, connecting body and mind. "Walking meditation makes us whole again. Only when we are connected with our body are we truly alive. Healing is not possible without that connection. So walk and breathe in such a way that you can connect with your body deeply."[8]

Here are two guided walking meditations to help you get started. Or use your favorite search engine to find your own. Again, some online apps mentioned previously provide access to guided walking meditations as well, both free and for purchase.

- Thich Nhat Hanh – Walking Meditation (6 minutes): https://www.youtube.com/watch?v=QdOIvZJgUu0
- Jack Kornfield – Walking Meditation (5 ½ minutes): https://jackkornfield.com/walking-meditation-2/

ENHANCE YOUR PRACTICE

Once you've had a chance to practice meditating in nature, either still or walking, make it happen more often if you love it. Get your calendar out and schedule your time in nature. Make it a non-negotiable date. You may want to share this date with someone you know who would enjoy and benefit from it. Silent walking in nature with another can be a very deep, shared experience.

❧ 6 ❧

MEDITATE WITH GRATITUDE

I choose to notice and express gratitude

for the sight of moonlight,

the sounds of laughter and birdsong,

the flavor of a nourishing meal,

and the chance to walk and breathe in the woods.

I acknowledge the often-silent beauty of life,

and the many reasons to give thanks. – TM

Gratitude (noun) – "a strong feeling of appreciation to someone or something for what the person has done to help you; the feeling or quality of being grateful."[1]

Most of us understand the meaning of gratitude, being thankful or appreciative of something someone says or does.

At times, gratitude arises automatically when we are the recipient of a kind act, such as someone holding a door open for us, or letting us go ahead of them in the grocery line when we only have one or two items and they have a full cart.

We may automatically say "thank you" when someone blesses us after a sneeze or pays a compliment. True gratitude can be as simple as noticing when these common courtesies are offered, instead of saying the words "thank you" without even thinking, say them with the true intention of giving thanks. It all comes back to noticing and acting with intention.

When we take a moment to give thanks for something, we actually begin to notice more good things around us, more opportunities for gratitude. Ever notice the colors of the sunset on the drive home from a stressful day at work and how you then start finding other reasons to calm down and smile? Your partner, kids, or dog welcoming you home becomes that much sweeter if you've already broken the negativity from your day by saying "thank you" for something beautiful on the way home. There's a definite domino effect when it comes to practicing gratitude.

BENEFITS OF PRACTICING GRATITUDE

Feeling gratitude on a regular basis can literally transform your life. By focusing on what you *have* instead of what you lack, or finding what's good in a person or situation instead of complaining or getting caught up in the drama as your default reaction, your overall satisfaction with life increases. An article from the Yale Center for Emotional Intelligence states that, "Grateful people experience more joy, love, and enthusiasm, and they enjoy protection from destructive emotions like envy, greed, and bitterness."[2]

Some of the other known benefits of practicing gratitude include:

- reduced stress
- making new friends – people are more likely to continue the conversation with someone who has acknowledged their act of kindness[3]
- improved physical health – reduced aches and pains, increased feelings of better overall health[4]
- increased happiness[5]
- reduced depression
- increased sensitivity and empathy toward others
- better sleep – a study of 401 people with clinically impaired sleep showed that "more grateful people reported falling asleep more quickly, sleeping longer, having better sleep quality, and staying awake more easily during the day."[6]
- improved self-esteem – helping others makes you feel better about yourself
- increased resilience to better handle challenging or traumatic events

One study considered the effect of gratitude journaling in almost 300 people with existing mental health issues. The findings suggest that "gratitude writing can be beneficial not just for healthy, well-adjusted individuals, but also for those who struggle with mental health concerns. In fact, it seems, practicing gratitude on top of receiving psychological counseling carries greater benefits than counseling alone, even when that gratitude practice is brief."[7]

FINDING AND EXPRESSING GRATITUDE

There are many ways to give thanks for the special moments in each day. But first comes the noticing, the awareness of those subtle parts of life that are indeed amazing and wonderful. Often the only noticed moments are the ones when something goes wrong. Taking the time to notice what went right is a good habit to create.

My friend, Gene, tells the story of having to walk up 73 steps to get to his apartment. In all the time he lived there, going up and down the stairs multiple times each day, he only noticed two of those 73-step journeys. Both of them were when he tripped going up. He didn't remember any of the safe journeys. What if, instead, each safe journey was noticed and appreciated as a victory? What if the practice of noticing and appreciating was carried through the whole day?

A helpful way to start the practice of noticing is by taking time for a quick gratitude meditation. Five minutes in stillness to replay your day, paying particular attention to the positive parts, can yield surprising results. Not only will you feel better after those five minutes, your practice of noticing the good will expand. You'll enjoy more and more moments as you encounter them. And when you practice taking two seconds to say "thank you" either silently or out loud, you invite more good into your life.

What might you notice that is worthy of gratitude? The list is as long as each day and, even then, there's still more:

> waking up (that's an excellent start); having safe shelter; having the time, space, motivation and intention to meditate; having enough food; being warm (or cool) enough; being dry; hugs; hearing; seeing; tasting; being

able to walk or maneuver a wheelchair; smiling; having friends and/or family; hugs; the colors of sunrise and sunset; the sounds of birdsong and laughter; the smell of coffee brewing; having a car; having your car start when you need it; finding a good parking space; getting a job; leaving a job that's not right for you; getting a raise; hugs; 2-for-1 avocados; fresh tomatoes from the garden; toast; running water (maybe even warm water); the shade of a tree on a hot day; a blanket when it's cold; music; art; books; plays; rivers; oceans; the smell of salty breezes; hugs; light; (comfortable) furniture; awareness; a bed to sleep in; a pillow for your head; a chance to close your eyes and rest; sleep; waking up...

This short list came from less than five minutes of thinking. And yes, I enjoy and am grateful for hugs. I know you'll think of and notice more things for which you can be grateful, including people, places, events, and things that have meaning for you. The act of noticing will lift you up. Try it now...

In addition to the many times in each day that are waiting to be noticed and appreciated, I especially like to be still as I retire for the night. I recall my day and write down at least three things for which I am grateful. I've kept a gratitude journal with daily entries for about ten years now. At first, it was a physical notebook. With downsizing and travel, it has become an electronic version. Going to sleep with a grateful heart makes a huge difference in life.

William Arthur Ward put it well, "Feeling gratitude and not expressing it is like wrapping a present and not giving it."[8]

There are fun ways to express gratitude. In addition to saying "thank you" silently or out loud or keeping a gratitude journal, notice if someone goes that extra step for you. Make the effort to connect with them and verbally express your thanks. If a stranger holds a door for you, make eye contact and say, "thank you." If it's a friend or family member who has helped, you can send a card or treat them to lunch or coffee.

Gratitude can be shown with a smile or a return kindness. Noticing how good it feels when someone lets you merge in traffic may encourage you to behave in a similar manner toward others.

By consciously choosing not to complain in an inconvenient situation and, instead, focusing on something positive, you will turn the situation around not only for yourself, but for those around you. It's a gift to everyone involved when you don't add to the negative energy by being grumpy.[9]

A few ideas for expressing gratitude to the people in your life who love you include telling them about what they did that made your life better or giving a genuine longer-than-normal hug (if hugging is your thing and theirs as well). For those challenging people in your life, double-up on your patience and tolerance. Resist the urge to criticize or jump to conclusions about current or future interactions based on how things have gone in the past.[10]

Gratitude is a habit that I choose. This practice brings more and more good things into my life as I choose to show gratitude for what is. There is always something for which to be thankful, regardless of the situation. Take a breath, be still, look around, and allow yourself to find it.

Giving thanks... it's a simple act that will turn your attitude around in a heartbeat and change your life for the better.

Here are a few free guided gratitude meditations to help you get started, or you can use your favorite search engine to find your own.

- Gratitude Meditation from Greater Good in Action at Berkeley University (10 minutes): https://ggia.berkeley.edu/practice/gratitude_meditation
- Guided Meditation on Gratitude and Forgiveness with Deepak Chopra (about 6 ½ minutes) https://www.youtube.com/watch?v=mUGMfyLXuhI
- Gratitude Meditation (Strengthen Happiness) from Stop, Breathe & Think (5 ½ minutes): https://www.youtube.com/watch?v=UhF8vLesRRc

ENHANCE YOUR PRACTICE

Try setting your watch to vibrate or set a timer to chime every hour during the most stressful parts of your day. When prompted, look up and around you and find five things for which you are thankful. Say them to yourself or out loud if you like. Some days and situations may require more effort, and that's exactly the time to practice because that's when you need it most. Smile when you notice your practice gets easier.

❧ 7 ❧

YOGA NIDRA MEDITATION

Settling into quiet stillness,

I am thankful for a chance

to notice, to recharge, to rest.

Settling into awareness

of breathing and sensations.

Nonreactive.

Only active witnessing.

The silent observer

learning to be with what is. – TM

Chronic stress impacts both the quantity and quality of your sleep. In this chapter, you'll expand your meditation practice with a method that provides the benefits of deep sleep, helping you break the cycle of "too stressed to sleep and too tired to get anything done so I'm stressed."

You'll find this new meditation easy and enjoyable. All you have to do is make the time for yourself to lie comfortably still and listen to a sequenced, guided relaxation session. With practice, you'll be able to relax deeply just by listening to these powerful meditations. And you'll continue to enjoy feeling relaxed, well-rested, and well-resourced for long after the meditation ends.

WHAT IS YOGA NIDRA?

Yoga nidra is a guided meditation that provides a systematic, progressive awareness of the body, breath, sensations, and emotions, which leads to profoundly deep rest and calm. I call it a power nap. Everyone, including children as young as three, can benefit from a guided yoga nidra session.

A yoga nidra meditation can be as short as five minutes or as long as sixty minutes or more, so you can choose a length based on the time you have available. Yoga nidra sessions are offered at yoga studios, workshops, or retreats, or as guided audios that you can listen to online or download. You don't need to practice yoga to practice yoga nidra, as it involves no movements at all.

Yoga nidra means "yogic sleep," and it's described as the deepest possible state of relaxation while still remaining conscious. You may feel like you're drifting in and out of sleep, and that's okay because you'll still benefit as your subconscious hears the words guiding you into this relaxed state of rest.

A yoga nidra meditation can be just as restorative as sleep. Used prior to your sleep time, it allows for a gentle slowing down and focusing of your mind, helping you to drift off more easily. All you need to do is get comfortable in your bed and listen to a guided session, using earphones if you like. As long as you're comfortable and able to be still, you'll benefit from this practice. More than once, I've awakened with the earphones still in my ears after an especially relaxing session!

BENEFITS OF YOGA NIDRA

Got stress? Yoga nidra calms, quiets, and brings clarity to the mind and body and allows for full-body relaxation.[1] It's even better than a typical mindfulness meditation for reducing stress. By giving the mind a continual moving focus during the progressive body and breath scan, the nervous system calms and stress levels decrease. Studies over the past four decades by Dr. Richard Miller, Rod Stryker, and many others have shown that a yoga nidra practice is beneficial for stress and post-traumatic stress disorder (PTSD).[2] As Rod Stryker points out, "We live in a chronically exhausted, overstimulated world."[3] Yoga nidra helps relieve the daily stress we face.

Suffer from sleep disorders? A 2016 randomized controlled study of individuals with sleep disorders showed that the yoga nidra meditation group experienced a significantly longer time asleep than the two control groups.[4] Easing into sleep after a yoga nidra session is something you need to experience to fully understand. You'll feel comforted and relaxed as you drift off to sleep more easily. Practicing yoga nidra also helps you fall back to sleep if you wake up in the middle of the night. Overcoming insomnia is a wonderful thing!

Anxious or depressed? A 2011 randomized controlled trial of 150 women showed that both anxiety and depression decreased significantly in the group that practiced yoga nidra. In addition, positive well-being, general health, and vitality improved significantly after six months of yoga nidra practice when compared with the control group who did not practice yoga nidra.[5]

Have trouble knowing what you want or need? A yoga nidra practice allows increased self-awareness. This practice brings you to a relaxed state, which can help you calmly recognize and acknowledge old stress response habits and create more helpful responses to those triggers. Awareness is the important first step. Making a better choice then becomes possible. We create new and better habits when we're aware of the old ones.

Want to keep that feeling of calm for longer? A regular practice of yoga nidra allows you to carry the calm and relaxed feeling you find during your practice back into your daily life, so your confident, creative brain can do its best. It allows you to feel more connected to self and others, which reduces stress by decreasing feelings of loneliness and separation.

HOW TO PRACTICE YOGA NIDRA MEDITATION

The best way to understand the benefits of yoga nidra is to try it. You can start with one of the free guided yoga nidra meditations offered below.

During this practice, you'll recline in a comfortable position, fully supported so you can rest without moving. You'll be gently guided through setting an intention for your session. As Dr. Miller describes, this intention could be a heartfelt desire you have and would like to see as truth, for yourself or for someone else. For example, learning to react to stress in a healthier way might be a heartfelt desire to set if that feels right for you. Or, think about something you'd like to achieve for yourself or to wish for someone else. Think big here if you like. I've had amazing results when I ask for what seems impossible.

Then you'll be guided through a brief awareness of the individual parts of the head and body followed by focusing awareness on the breath. You'll explore opposites of sensations, which definitely gives the busy mind something to focus on and teaches the ability to find the balanced center point between opposites. As the meditation nears its end, you'll revisit and reaffirm your intention before being guided to gently wake the body. A yoga nidra practice for sleep will not include the step to wake the body. This process is an amazing gift to yourself. It will reduce your stress, which will lead to feelings of complete relaxation, joy, well-being, connection, and peace.

When you're ready to expand your home yoga nidra meditation practice, there are several good, free apps for Android and iPhone such as Insight Timer (Dr. Miller has a solid presence on this app), Headspace, and Stop, Breathe & Think. You can also find other apps that require a fee to access, or even CDs for purchase. For group practices, check with local yoga studios or Meetup groups in your area.

Here are two more free online yoga nidra practices of varying length for you to experience:

- iRest® Yoga Nidra by Dr. Richard Miller (20 minutes): https://www.youtube.com/watch? v=Psl9FKh6qPg
- For deep relaxation to help you fall asleep by Yoga Journal (12 minutes): https://www.yogajournal.com/ videos/yoga-nidra-video-a-guided-practice-for-deep-relaxation

ENHANCE YOUR PRACTICE

Try practices from several different teachers to experience a range of lengths, voices, sounds, and areas of concentration. I highly recommend any of Dr. Miller's yoga nidra CDs as practice companions or his books for a deeper understanding of yoga nidra.[6] Choose several you like and set up a regular practice, perhaps weekly. I know your time is precious, and I believe once you've tried yoga nidra a few times, you'll agree that it deserves to be a priority in your self-care toolkit.

❧ 8 ❧

MAKING MEDITATION A HABIT FOR GOOD

Curiosity... how can they sit with serene faces,

in quiet stillness for so long,

gentle smiles of knowingness, radiating calm.

Curiosity... beckons to me now.

I am open to learning. – TM

This is the part where I turn it over to you. I've introduced different ways of starting a new meditation practice or expanding your existing practice. These methods may not all feel right for you, but I am confident you can find at least one to gracefully ease into your life.

If you truly wish to experience any of the many proven benefits that meditation provides, you need to make meditation a deliberate daily practice. You need to believe that you matter, because you do, and that you are worthy of setting aside some amount of time daily to improve the quality of your life.

If you're not sure that meditation is really going to make a difference in your life, can you commit yourself to try twenty-one days of a daily ten-minute meditation practice? Too much? Can you start by giving yourself just one minute each day? Then can you grow your practice one minute at a time until you reach ten minutes each day and see how that feels? You will probably find, once you commit to your practice, the time during your meditation flies by and you look forward to the next daily practice.

Can you identify any openings on your calendar where you can schedule time for yourself to be still and breathe, listen to a guided meditation, think about and write down the parts of your day for which you are thankful, spend time in nature, or walk with awareness?

Commitment to a new habit can be hard, especially if you're already feeling overwhelmed and stretched for time. But I promise a meditation practice is something that will pay you back with feelings of freedom and lightness. Meditation somehow makes you feel like you have more time along with less stress.

If you find yourself coming up with excuses for why you can't possibly take ten minutes for yourself each day, ask yourself how these excuses are helping you. What do you gain by not trying, by staying stuck? If you're still reading this, I believe you're ready to give it a try. See what happens. Practice and notice, because this is your chance to take care of yourself.

My friend Becky Watson, a gifted yoga therapist who also has a daily meditation practice, shares "When I'm consistent with my meditation, that's when I notice the biggest changes. It took me years to get to where I was consistent, but now that I'm in that place, *I have a hard time imagining life without my meditation practice.* Being consistent brings me a sense of being more centered and more connected to myself."[1]

~

ENHANCE YOUR PRACTICE

I recommend you take a few minutes now to make a plan for your daily meditation practice. Can you start today or tonight, even with one minute? Consider all the possible times in your life when you would be able to practice. Which method will you try first? Is there a meditation group somewhere nearby you could check out? When you're ready, practicing meditation with a group is powerful.

Choosing to start your daily meditation practice is a powerful, ongoing gift to yourself that keeps on giving. Daily meditation allows the possibility to notice small miracles while fully engaged in life's day-to-day activities and adventures. Practice patience and self-compassion when it comes to starting your practice. Don't give up if you miss a day. Try not to get frustrated if you get worried about doing it wrong. There is no wrong. Start again... as many times as it takes. You deserve this!

NOTES

Chapter 1 Guided Relaxation Meditation

1. Sign up to receive your **free guided relaxation meditation audio** download at https://fromstressedtocalm.com/restnow/

Chapter 2 Why Meditate?

1. Meditation https://www.merriam-webster.com/dictionary/meditation
2. Meditation https://www.yogapedia.com/definition/4949/meditation
3. Meditation https://dictionary.cambridge.org/dictionary/english/meditation
4. A comparison of mindfulness-based stress reduction and an active control in modulation of neurogenic inflammation https://www.sciencedirect.com/science/article/pii/S0889159112004758
5. Effects of the transcendental meditation technique on trait anxiety: a meta-analysis of randomized

controlled trials https://www.ncbi.nlm.nih.gov/pubmed/24107199

6. Mindfulness-Based Stress Reduction for Health Care Professionals: Results from a Randomized Trial http://psycnet.apa.org/record/2005-05099-004

7. Mind the Trap: Mindfulness Practice Reduces Cognitive Rigidity http://journals.plos.org/plosone/article?id=10.1371/journal.pone.0036206

8. Mindfulness training modifies subsystems of attention https://link.springer.com/article/10.3758/CABN.7.2.109#page-1

9. Initial results from a study of the effects of meditation on multitasking performance https://dl.acm.org/citation.cfm?id=1979862

10. The value of mindfulness meditation in the treatment of insomnia https://www.ncbi.nlm.nih.gov/pubmed/26390335

11. Brain Mechanisms Supporting Modulation of Pain by Mindfulness Meditation https://www.ncbi.nlm.nih.gov/pmc/articles/PMC3090218/

12. Top 141 benefits of meditation, broken down by physical, mental, emotional, and spiritual benefits https://eocinstitute.org/meditation/141-benefits-of-meditation/

Chapter 3 Meditate on the Breath

1. For quick articles about the different sutras, see this Yoga Journal compilation https://www.yogajournal.com/yoga-101/philosophy/yoga-sutras

2. For more information about Vietnamese Buddhist monk Thich Nhat Hanh, see https://plumvillage.org/about/thich-nhat-hanh/

3. For more information, see the EOC Institute's

writings on meditation and the benefits of mindful breathing https://eocinstitute.org/meditation/meditation-and-breathing-benefits-of-mindful-breathing/

4. For more information, see https://www.drweil.com/health-wellness/body-mind-spirit/stress-anxiety/breathing-three-exercises/ for more information on the 4-7-8 Breath as well as two more breathing techniques for stress reduction

Chapter 4 Meditate with Kindness

1. For more from and about meditation expert Sharon Salzberg, see https://www.sharonsalzberg.com/

2. Greater Happiness in 5 Minutes a Day https://greatergood.berkeley.edu/article/item/better_than_sex_and_appropriate_for_kids

3. Science-Backed Reasons to Try Loving Kindness Meditation https://www.psychologytoday.com/us/blog/feeling-it/201409/18-science-backed-reasons-try-loving-kindness-meditation

4. Carson JW, Keefe FJ, Lynch TR, Carson KM, Goli V, Fras AM, Thorp SR, Loving-kindness meditation for chronic low back pain: results from a pilot trial, *Journal of Holistic Nursing* 2005, Sep; 23(3):287-304 https://www.ncbi.nlm.nih.gov/pubmed/16049118

5. University of Sussex. Seven minutes of meditation can reduce racial prejudice, study finds. *ScienceDaily*. 2015. Retrieved October 31, 2018 from https://www.sciencedaily.com/releases/2015/11/151119122244.htm

Chapter 5 Meditate in Nature

1. The Benefits of Meditation Out of Doors https://

totallymeditation.com/meditating-outside-the-benefits/

2. Why Meditating In Nature Is Easier https://www.yogajournal.com/meditation/natural-wonder

3. Why Outdoor Meditation is Good for Your Health https://www.ehe.health/blog/outdoor-meditation

4. Meditating Outside | Benefits & Joys of Meditating in Nature https://mindworks.org/blog/meditating-outside-nature/

5. Why Forest Bathing Is Good for Your Health https://greatergood.berkeley.edu/article/item/why_forest_bathing_is_good_for_your_health

6. Li, Qing, MD, Forest Bathing: How Trees Can Help You Find Health and Happiness, 2018 My Book

7. Walking Meditation https://ggia.berkeley.edu/practice/walking_meditation

8. Thich Nhat Hanh on Walking Meditation https://www.lionsroar.com/how-to-meditate-thich-nhat-hanh-on-walking-meditation/

Chapter 6 Meditate with Gratitude

1. Definition of gratitude from the Cambridge Dictionary https://dictionary.cambridge.org/us/dictionary/english/gratitude

2. Gratitude Practice Explained http://ei.yale.edu/what-is-gratitude/

3. 7 Scientifically Proven Benefits of Gratitude https://www.psychologytoday.com/us/blog/what-mentally-strong-people-dont-do/201504/7-scientifically-proven-benefits-gratitude

4. Berkeley studies on the health benefits of gratitude https://greatergood.berkeley.edu/article/item/is_gratitude_good_for_your_health

5. Summary of studies on gratitude and happiness https://www.health.harvard.edu/healthbeat/giving-thanks-can-make-you-happier

6. Wood, Alex M, Joseph, Stephen, Lloyd, Joanna, and Atkins, Samuel, Gratitude influences sleep through the mechanism of pre-sleep cognitions, *Journal of Psychosomatic Research* 66 (2009) 43–48, https://greatergood.berkeley.edu/images/application_uploads/Wood-GratitudeSleep.pdf

7. How Gratitude Changes You and Your Brain https://greatergood.berkeley.edu/article/item/how_gratitude_changes_you_and_your_brain

8. William Arthur Ward Quotes https://www.brainyquote.com/authors/william-arthur-ward-quotes

9. 5 Simple Ways to Express Gratitude Every Day https://www.entrepreneur.com/article/235785

10. 50 Ways to Show Gratitude for the People in Your Life https://tinybuddha.com/blog/50-ways-to-show-gratitude-for-the-people-in-your-life/

Chapter 7 Yoga Nidra Meditation

1. Yoga Nidra: Systematic Meditation https://yogainternational.com/article/view/5-benefits-of-yoga-nidra

2. For more information about Integrative Restoration (iRest®) and Dr. Richard Miller, see https://www.irest.org/

3. Rod Stryker, founder of ParaYoga https://www.parayoga.com/rod-stryker/

4. For more information see "Comparative Effectiveness of Three Occupational Therapy Sleep Interventions: A Randomized Controlled Study."

https://www.irest.us/sites/default/files/
Sleep_Interventions_Study_Pub_16.pdf

5. For more information see "Impact of *Yoga Nidra* on psychological general wellbeing in patients with menstrual irregularities: A randomized controlled trial." https://www.ncbi.nlm.nih.gov/pmc/articles/PMC3099097/

6. Popular Products by Dr. Richard Miller https://www.irest.org/irest-yoga-nidra-meditation-products

Chapter 8 Making Meditation a Habit for Good

1. Don't Neglect Your Meditation Practice https://www.beckywatsonyoga.com/2019/dont-neglect-your-meditation-practice/

ACKNOWLEDGMENTS

Many thanks to my village:

Thank you, Deb Maluk, for your dedication to your art of photography even in the wee hours and crazy-low temperatures of Manitoba, Canada. I'm so happy to have your beautiful works on the covers in this series.

Thank you, Jill McBurney, for being a mentor from the first day I met you. Your editing skills make this a better book and your compassion and guidance as a yoga teacher give me tools to use and share.

Thank you, Diana Needham and your Team for transforming Deb's beautiful pictures into awesome and inspirational book covers.

Thank you, Family and Friends, for being You.

A SPECIAL REQUEST

If you loved this book, please leave an honest review where you purchased it. By leaving a review, you help search engines show this book to more readers. Thank you so much for your support!

ABOUT THE AUTHOR

Terry Maluk is a gifted stress-management coach and author of multiple bestselling books that provide methods for learning to reduce stress and rediscover joy. A member of the American Holistic Nurses Association, Terry holds a Master of Science degree in Public Health, is an accredited, certified Emotional Freedom Techniques (EFT Tapping) practitioner, and a registered yoga teacher. Her extensive experience and her passion for helping others make her books excellent resources for anyone ready to start their journey toward a happier life.

FromStressedToCalm.com

Made in the USA
Columbia, SC
16 January 2020

87047725R00046